The Ultimate Way to Diabetic Diet for Busy People

Do Not Waste Your Time to Get Back in Shape and Make Healthy Smoothies

Danielle Woods

contained within this document, including, but not limited to, —
errors, omissions, or inaccuracies.

Table of contents

Peach & Apricot Smoothie

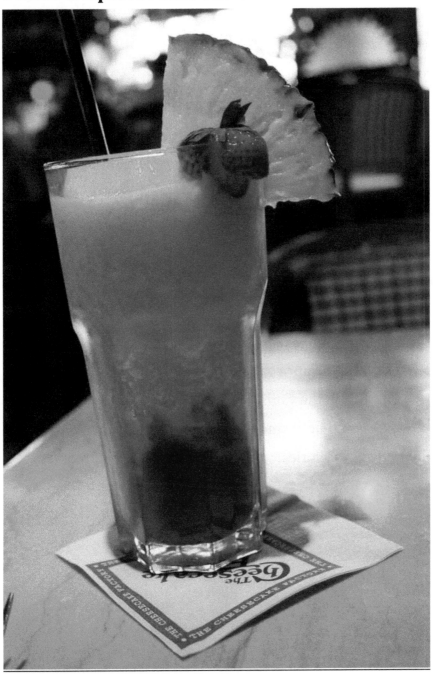

Preparation Time : 11 minutes

Cooking Time : 0 minute

Serving : 2

Ingredients :

- 1 cup almond milk (unsweetened)
- 1 teaspoon honey
- ½ cup apricots, sliced
- ½ cup peaches, sliced
- ½ cup carrot, chopped
- 1 teaspoon vanilla extract

Directions :

1. Mix milk and honey.
2. Pour into a blender.
3. Add the apricots, peaches and carrots.
4. Stir in the vanilla.
5. Blend until smooth.

Nutrition : 153 Calories; 30g Carbohydrate; 32.6g Protein

Tropical Smoothie

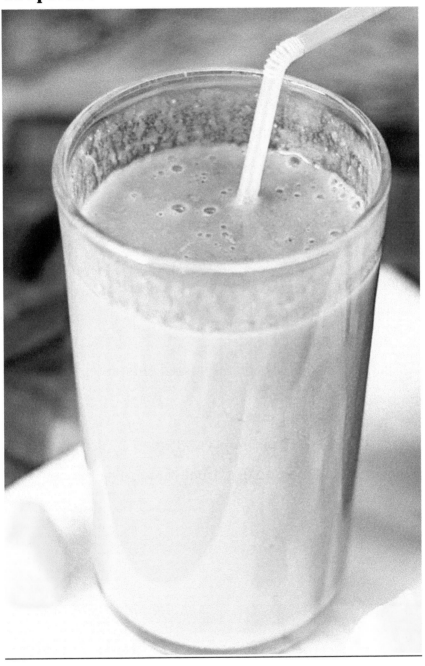

Preparation Time : 8 minutes

Cooking Time : 0 minute

Serving : 2

Ingredients :

- 1 banana, sliced
- 1 cup mango, sliced
- 1 cup pineapple, sliced
- 1 cup peaches, sliced
- 6 oz. nonfat coconut yogurt
- Pineapple wedges

Directions :

1. Freeze the fruit slices for 1 hour.
2. Transfer to a blender.
3. Stir in the rest of the ingredients except pineapple wedges.
4. Process until smooth.
5. Garnish with pineapple wedges.

Nutrition : 102 Calories; 22.6g Carbohydrate; 2.5g Protein

Banana & Strawberry Smoothie

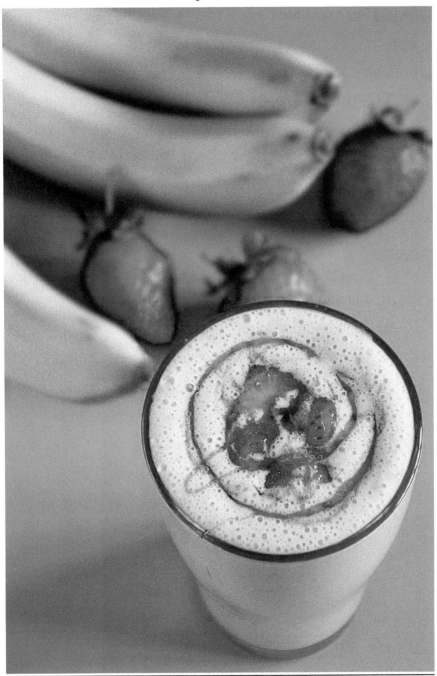

Preparation Time : 7 minutes

Cooking Time : 0 minute

Serving : 2

Ingredients :

- 1 banana, sliced
- 4 cups fresh strawberries, sliced
- 1 cup ice cubes
- 6 oz. yogurt
- 1 kiwi fruit, sliced

Directions :

1. Add banana, strawberries, ice cubes and yogurt in a blender.
2. Blend until smooth.
3. Garnish with kiwi fruit slices and serve.

Nutrition : 54 Calories; 11.8g Carbohydrate; 1.7g Protein

Cantaloupe & Papaya Smoothie

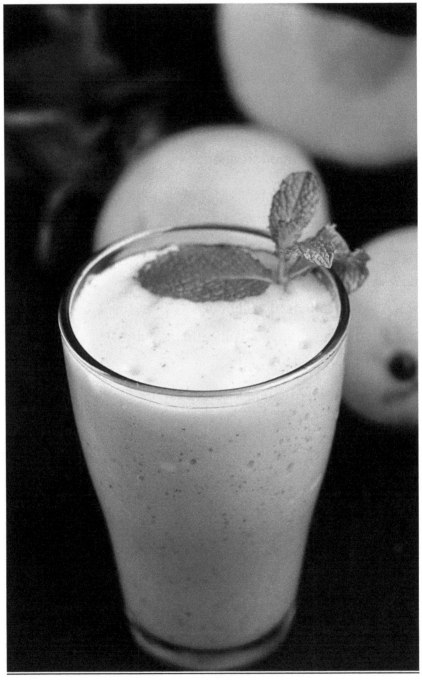

Preparation Time : 9 minutes

Cooking Time : 0 minute

Serving : 2

Ingredients :

- ¾ cup low-fat milk
- ½ cup papaya, chopped
- ½ cup cantaloupe, chopped
- ½ cup mango, cubed
- 4 ice cubes
- Lime zest

Directions :

1. Pour milk into a blender.
2. Add the chopped fruits and ice cubes.
3. Blend until smooth.
4. Garnish with lime zest and serve.

Nutrition : 207 Calories; 18.4g Carbohydrate; 7.7g Protein

Watermelon & Cantaloupe Smoothie

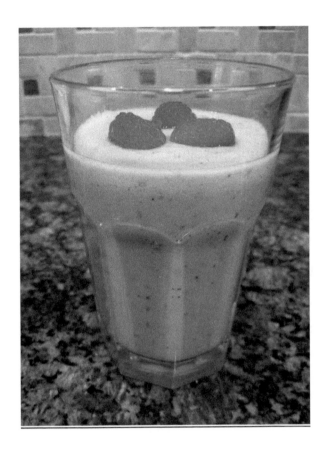

Preparation Time : 10 minutes

Cooking Time : 0 minute

Serving : 2

Ingredients :

- 2 cups watermelon, sliced
- 1 cup cantaloupe, sliced
- ½ cup nonfat yogurt
- ¼ cup orange juice

Directions :

1. Add all the ingredients to a blender.

2. Blend until creamy and smooth.

3. Chill before serving.

Nutrition : 114 Calories; 13g Carbohydrate; 4.8g Protein

Raspberry and Peanut Butter Smoothie

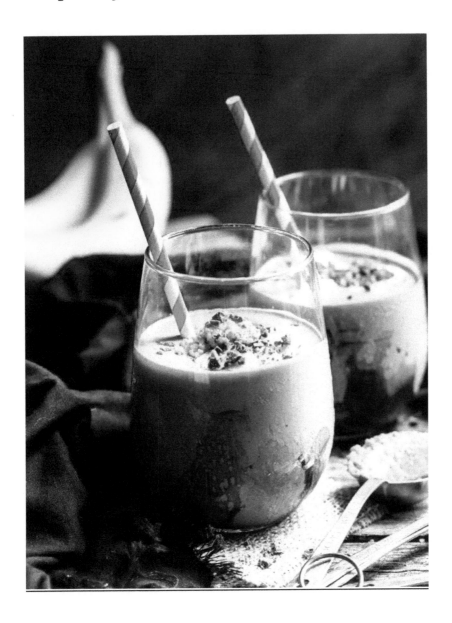

Preparation Time : 10 minutes

Cooking Time : 0 minute

Serving : 2

Ingredients :

- Peanut butter, smooth and natural [2 tbsp]
- Skim milk [2 tbsp]
- Raspberries, fresh [1 or 1 ½ cups]
- Ice cubes [1 cup]
- Stevia [2 tsp]

Directions :

1. Situate all the ingredients in your blender. Set the mixer to puree. Serve.

Nutrition : 170 Calories; 8.6g Fat; 20g Carbohydrate

Strawberry, Kale and Ginger Smoothie

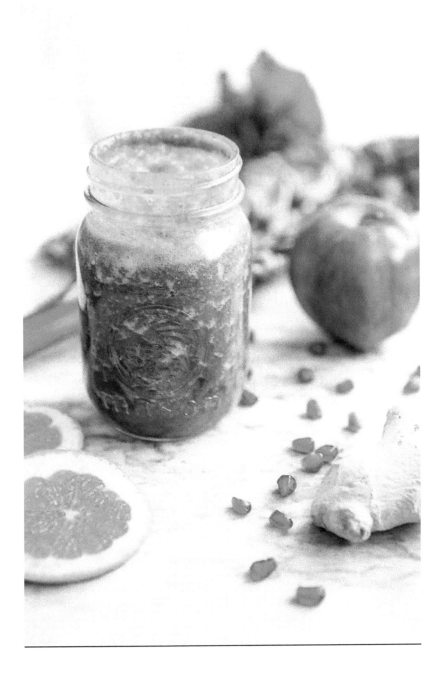

Preparation Time : 13 minutes

Cooking Time : 0 minute

Serving : 2

Ingredients :

- Curly kale leaves, fresh and large with stems removed [6 pcs]
- Grated ginger, raw and peeled [2 tsp]
- Water, cold [½ cup]
- Lime juice [3 tbsp]
- Honey [2 tsp]
- Strawberries, fresh and trimmed [1 or 1 ½ cups]
- Ice cubes [1 cup]

Directions :

1. Position all the ingredients in your blender. Set to puree. Serve.

Nutrition : 205 Calories; 2.9g Fat; 42.4g Carbohydrates

Berry Mint Smoothie

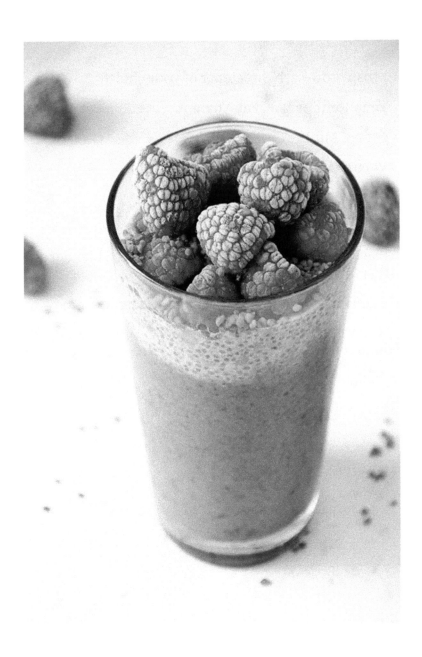

Preparation Time : 5 Minutes

Cooking Time : 5 Minutes

Servings : 2

Ingredients :

- 1 tbsp. Low-carb Sweetener of your choice
- 1 cup Kefir or Low Fat-Yoghurt
- 2 tbsp. Mint
- ¼ cup Orange
- 1 cup Mixed Berries

Directions :

1. Place all of the ingredients in a high-speed blender and then blend it until smooth.
2. Transfer the smoothie to a serving glass and enjoy it.

Nutrition : Calories: 137Kcal; Carbohydrates: 11g; Proteins: 6g; Fat: 1g; Sodium: 64mg

Greenie Smoothie

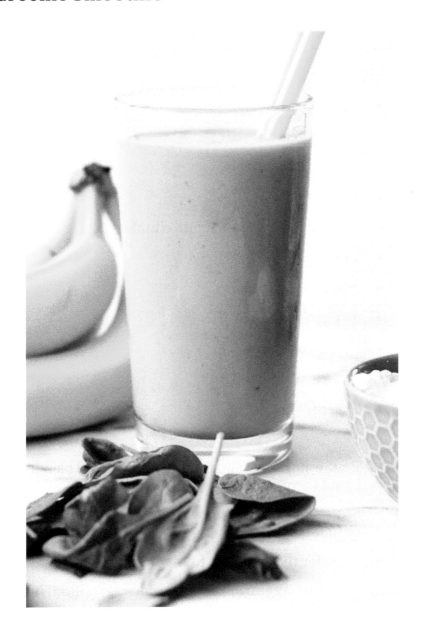

Preparation Time : 5 Minutes

Cooking Time : 5 Minutes

Servings : 2

Ingredients :

- 1 1/2 cup Water
- 1 tsp. Stevia
- 1 Green Apple, ripe
- 1 tsp. Stevia
- 1 Green Pear, chopped into chunks
- 1 Lime
- 2 cups Kale, fresh
- ¾ tsp. Cinnamon
- 12 Ice Cubes
- 20 Green Grapes
- 1/2 cup Mint, fresh

Directions :

1. Pour water, kale, and pear in a high-speed blender and blend them for 2 to 3 minutes until mixed.
2. Stir in all the remaining ingredients into it and blend until it becomes smooth.
3. Transfer the smoothie to serving glass.

Nutrition : Calories: 123Kcal; Carbohydrates: 27g; Proteins: 2g; Fat: 2g; Sodium: 30mg

Coconut Spinach Smoothie

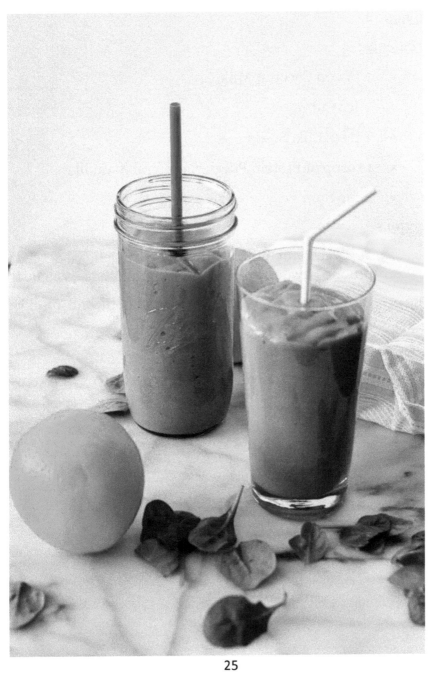

Preparation Time : 5 Minutes

Cooking Time : 5 Minutes

Servings : 2

Ingredients :

- 1 ¼ cup Coconut Milk
- 2 Ice Cubes
- 2 tbsp. Chia Seeds
- 1 scoop of Protein Powder, preferably vanilla
- 1 cup Spin

Directions :

1. Pour coconut milk along with spinach, chia seeds, protein powder, and ice cubes in a high-speed blender.
2. Blend for 2 minutes to get a smooth and luscious smoothie.
3. Serve in a glass and enjoy it.

Nutrition : Calories: 251Kcal; Carbohydrates: 10.9g; Proteins: 20.3g; Fat: 15.1g; Sodium: 102mg

Oats Coffee Smoothie

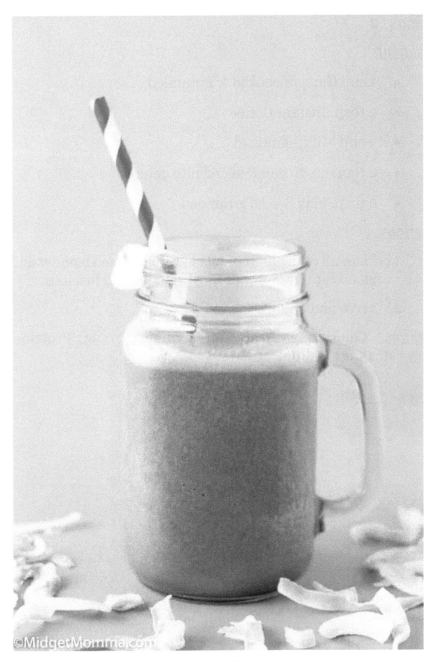

Preparation Time : 5 Minutes

Cooking Time : 5 Minutes

Servings : 2

Ingredients :

- 1 cup Oats, uncooked & grounded
- 2 tbsp. Instant Coffee
- 3 cup Milk, skimmed
- 2 Banana, frozen & sliced into chunks
- 2 tbsp. Flax Seeds, grounded

Directions :

1. Place all of the ingredients in a high-speed blender and blend for 2 minutes or until smooth and luscious.
2. Serve and enjoy.

Nutrition : Calories: 251Kcal; Carbohydrates: 10.9g; Proteins: 20.3g; Fat: 15.1g; Sodium: 102mg

Veggie Smoothie

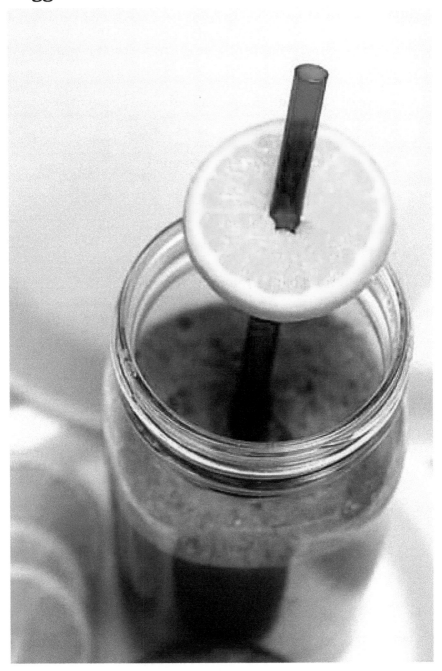

Preparation Time : 5 Minutes

Cooking Time : 5 Minutes

Servings : 1

Ingredients :

- ¼ of 1 Red Bell Pepper, sliced
- 1/2 tbsp. Coconut Oil
- 1 cup Almond Milk, unsweetened
- ¼ tsp. Turmeric
- 4 Strawberries, chopped
- Pinch of Cinnamon
- 1/2 of 1 Banana, preferably frozen

Directions :

1. Combine all the ingredients required to make the smoothie in a high-speed blender.
2. Blend for 3 minutes to get a smooth and silky mixture.
3. Serve and enjoy.

Nutrition : Calories: 169cal; Carbohydrates: 17g; Proteins: 2.3g; Fat: 9.8g; Sodium: 162mg

Avocado Smoothie

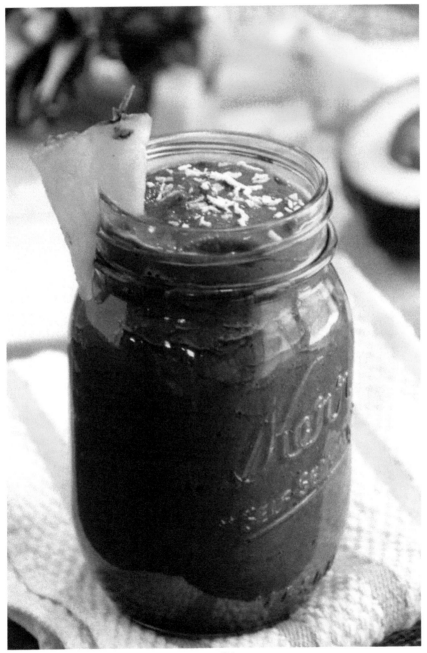

Preparation Time : 10 Minutes

Cooking Time : 0 Minutes

Servings : 2

Ingredients :

- 1 Avocado, ripe & pit removed
- 2 cups Baby Spinach
- 2 cups Water
- 1 cup Baby Kale
- 1 tbsp. Lemon Juice
- 2 sprigs of Mint
- 1/2 cup Ice Cubes

Directions :

1. Place all the ingredients needed to make the smoothie in a high-speed blender then blend until smooth.
2. Transfer to a serving glass and enjoy it.

Nutrition : Calories: 214cal; Carbohydrates: 15g; Proteins: 2g; Fat: 17g; Sodium: 25mg

Orange Carrot Smoothie

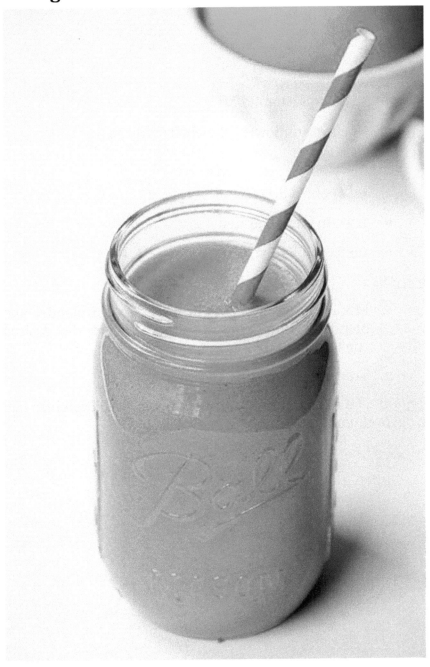

Preparation Time : 5 Minutes

Cooking Time : 0 Minutes

Servings : 1

Ingredients :

- 1 1/2 cups Almond Milk
- ¼ cup Cauliflower, blanched & frozen
- 1 Orange
- 1 tbsp. Flax Seed
- 1/3 cup Carrot, grated
- 1 tsp. Vanilla Extract

Directions :

1. Mix all the ingredients in a high-speed blender and blend for 2 minutes or until you get the desired consistency.

2. Transfer to a serving glass and enjoy it.

Nutrition : Calories: 216cal; Carbohydrates: 10g; Proteins: 15g; Fat: 7g; Sodium: 25mg

Blackberry Smoothie

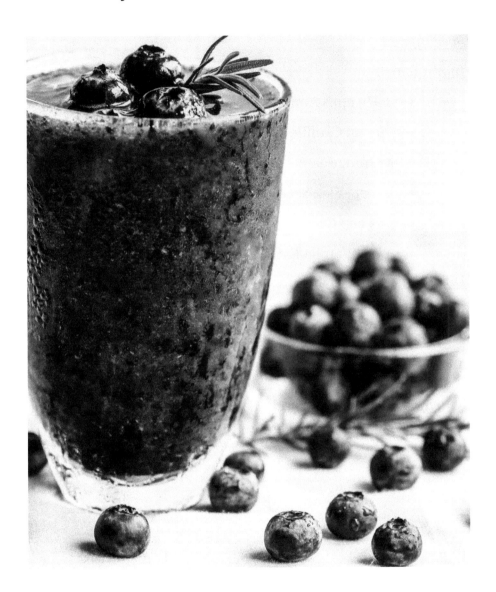

Preparation Time : 5 Minutes

Cooking Time : 0 Minutes

Servings : 1

Ingredients :

- 1 1/2 cups Almond Milk
- ¼ cup Cauliflower, blanched & frozen
- 1 Orange
- 1 tbsp. Flax Seed
- 1/3 cup Carrot, grated
- 1 tsp. Vanilla Extract

Directions :

1. Place all the ingredients needed to make the blackberry smoothie in a high-speed blender and blend for 2 minutes until you get a smooth mixture.

2. Transfer to a serving glass and enjoy it.

Nutrition : Calories: 275cal; Carbohydrates: 9g; Proteins: 11g; Fat: 17g; Sodium: 73mg

Key Lime Pie Smoothie

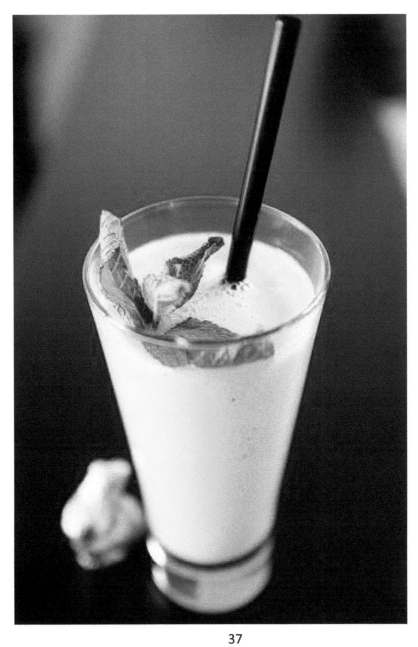

Preparation Time : 5 Minutes

Cooking Time : 0 Minutes

Servings : 1

Ingredients :

- 1/2 cup Cottage Cheese
- 1 tbsp. Sweetener of your choice
- 1/2 cup Water
- 1/2 cup Spinach
- 1 tbsp. Lime Juice
- 1 cup Ice Cubes

Directions :

1. Spoon in the ingredients to a high-speed blender and blend until silky smooth.
2. Transfer to a serving glass and enjoy it.

Nutrition : Calories: 180cal; Carbohydrates: 7g; Proteins: 36g; Fat: 1g; Sodium: 35mg

Cinnamon Roll Smoothie

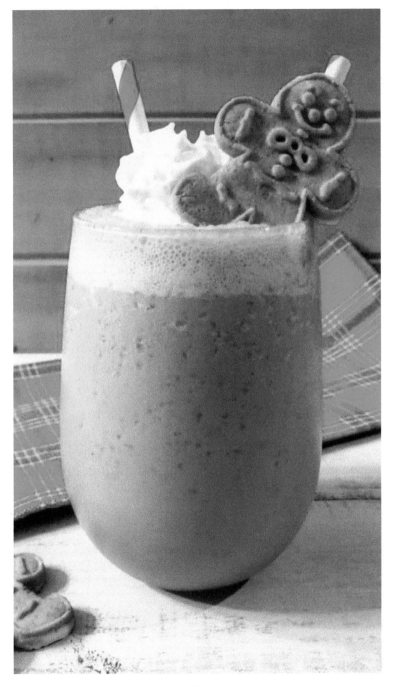

Preparation Time : 5 Minutes

Cooking Time : 0 Minutes

Servings : 1

Ingredients :

- 1 tsp. Flax Meal or oats, if preferred
- 1 cup Almond Milk
- 1/2 tsp. Cinnamon
- 2 tbsp. Protein Powder
- 1 cup Ice
- ¼ tsp. Vanilla Extract
- 4 tsp. Sweetener of your choice

Directions :

1. Pour the milk into the blender, followed by the protein powder, sweetener, flax meal, cinnamon, vanilla extract, and ice.
2. Blend for 40 seconds or until smooth.
3. Serve and enjoy.

Nutrition : Calories: 145cal; Carbohydrates: 1.6g; Proteins: 26.5g; Fat: 3.25g; Sodium: 30mg

Strawberry Cheesecake Smoothie

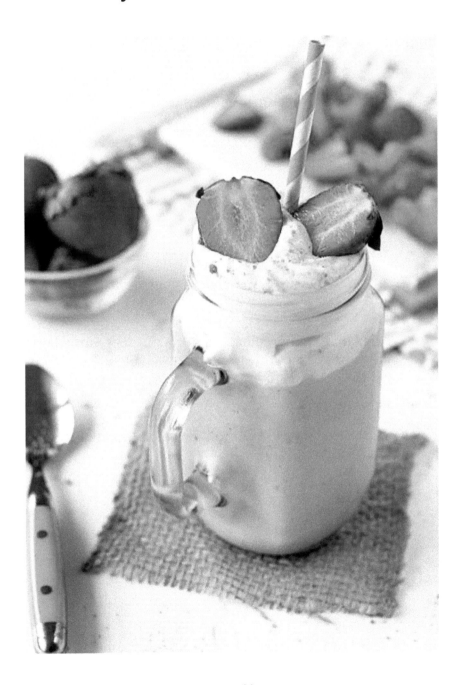

Preparation Time : 5 Minutes

Cooking Time : 0 Minutes

Servings : 1

Ingredients :

- ¼ cup Soy Milk, unsweetened
- 1/2 cup Cottage Cheese, low-fat
- 1/2 tsp. Vanilla Extract
- 2 oz. Cream Cheese
- 1 cup Ice Cubes
- 1/2 cup Strawberries
- 4 tbsp. Low-carb Sweetener of your choice

Directions :

1. Add all the ingredients for making the strawberry cheesecake smoothie to a high-speed blender until you get the desired smooth consistency.

2. Serve and enjoy.

Nutrition : Calories: 347cal; Carbohydrates: 10.05g; Proteins: 17.5g; Fat: 24g; Sodium: 45mg

Peanut Butter Banana Smoothie

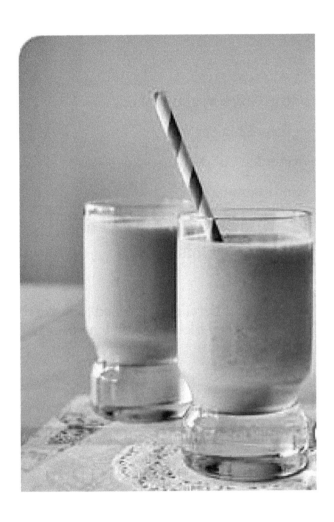

Preparation Time : 5 Minutes

Cooking Time : 2 Minutes

Servings : 1

Ingredients :

- ¼ cup Greek Yoghurt, plain
- ½ tbsp. Chia Seeds
- ½ cup Ice Cubes
- ½ of 1 Banana
- ½ cup Water
- 1 tbsp. Peanut Butter

Directions :

1. Place all the ingredients needed to make the smoothie in a high-speed blender and blend to get a smooth and luscious mixture.

2. Transfer the smoothie to a serving glass and enjoy it.

Nutrition : Calories: 202cal; Carbohydrates: 14g; Proteins: 10g; Fat: 9g; Sodium: 30mg

Avocado Turmeric Smoothie

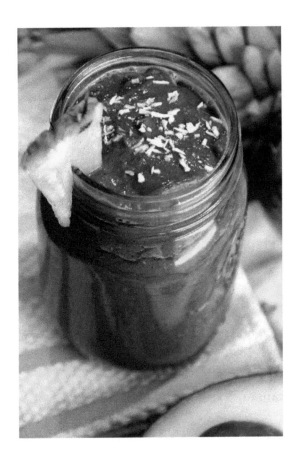

Preparation Time : 5 Minutes

Cooking Time : 2 Minutes

Servings : 1

Ingredients :

- 1/2 of 1 Avocado
- 1 cup Ice, crushed
- ¾ cup Coconut Milk, full-fat
- 1 tsp. Lemon Juice
- ¼ cup Almond Milk
- 1/2 tsp. Turmeric
- 1 tsp. Ginger, freshly grated

Directions :

1. Place all the ingredients excluding the crushed ice in a high-speed blender and blend for 2 to 3 minutes or until smooth.

2. Transfer to a serving glass and enjoy it.

Nutrition : Calories: 232cal; Carbohydrates: 4.1g; Proteins: 1.7g; Fat: 22.4g; Sodium: 25mg

Lemon Blueberry Smoothie

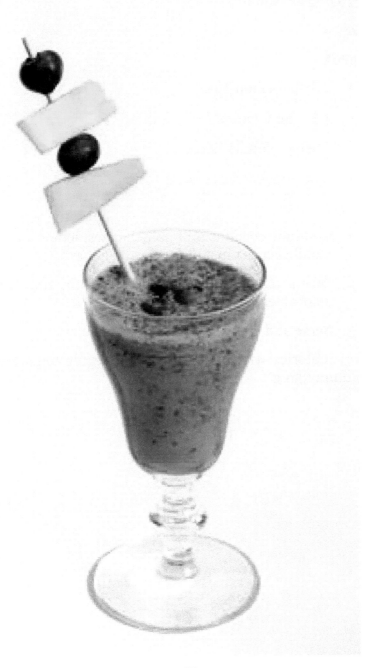

Preparation Time : 5 Minutes

Cooking Time : 2 Minutes

Servings : 2

Ingredients :

- 1 tbsp. Lemon Juice
- 1 ¾ cup Coconut Milk, full-fat
- 1/2 tsp. Vanilla Extract
- 3 oz. Blueberries, frozen

Directions :

1. Combine coconut milk, blueberries, lemon juice, and vanilla extract in a high-speed blender.
2. Blend for 2 minutes for a smooth and luscious smoothie.
3. Serve and enjoy.

Nutrition : Calories: 417cal; Carbohydrates: 9g;Proteins: 4g; Fat: 43g; Sodium: 35mg

Matcha Green Smoothie

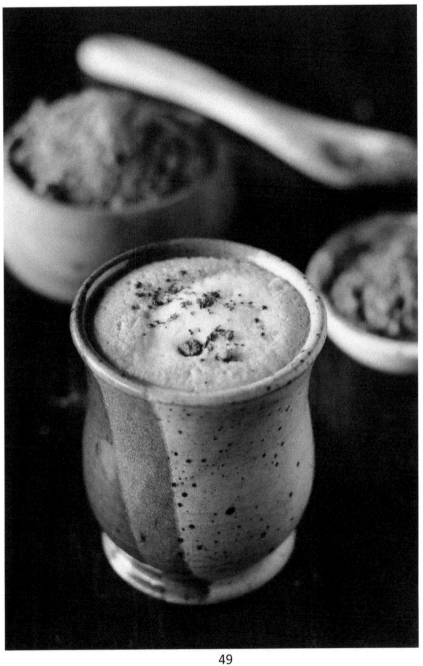

Preparation Time : 5 Minutes

Cooking Time : 2 Minutes

Servings : 2

Ingredients :

- ¼ cup Heavy Whipping Cream
- 1/2 tsp. Vanilla Extract
- 1 tsp. Matcha Green Tea Powder
- 2 tbsp. Protein Powder
- 1 tbsp. Hot Water
- 1 ¼ cup Almond Milk, unsweetened
- 1/2 of 1 Avocado, medium

Directions :

1. Place all the ingredients in the high-blender for one to two minutes.
2. Serve and enjoy.

Nutrition : Calories: 229cal; Carbohydrates: 1.5g; Proteins: 14.1g; Fat: 43g; Sodium: 35mg

Blueberry Smoothie

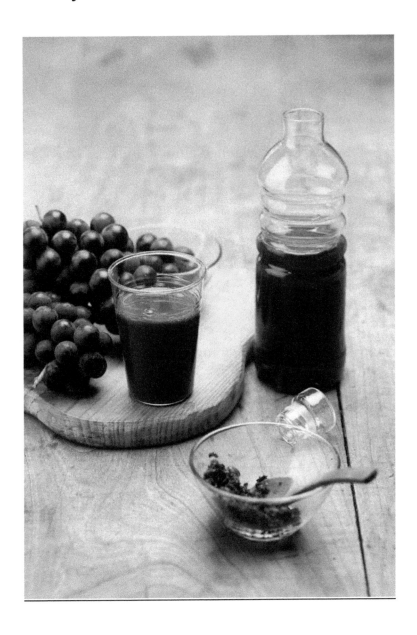

Preparation   Time   :   10   minutes
Cooking Time : 0 minutes

Servings : 2

Ingredients :

- 2 cups frozen blueberries

- 1 small banana

- 1½ cups unsweetened almond milk

- ¼ cup ice cubes

Directions :

1. Place all the ingredients in a high-speed blender and pulse until creamy.

2. Pour the smoothie into two glasses and serve immediately.

Nutrition : Calories 158; Total Fat 3.3 g; Saturated Fat 0.3 g; Cholesterol 0 mg; Sodium 137 mg; Total Carbs 34 g; Fiber 5.6 g; Sugar 20.6 g; Protein 2.4 g

Beet & Strawberry Smoothie

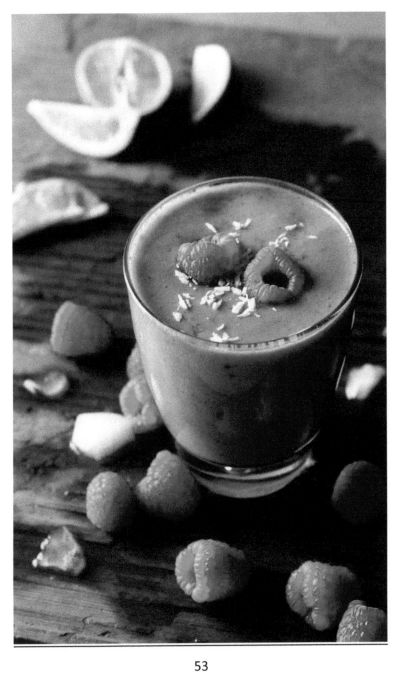

Preparation Time : 10 minutes
  Cooking Time : 0 minutes

Servings : 2

Ingredients :

- 2 cups frozen strawberries, pitted and chopped
- 2/3 cup roasted and frozen beet, chopped
- 1 teaspoon fresh ginger, peeled and grated
- 1 teaspoon fresh turmeric, peeled and grated
- ½ cup fresh orange juice
- 1 cup unsweetened almond milk

Directions :

1. Place all the ingredients in a high-speed blender and pulse until creamy.

2. Pour the smoothie into two glasses and serve immediately.

Nutrition : Calories 258; Total Fat 1.5 g; Saturated Fat 0.1 g; Cholesterol 0 mg; Sodium 134 mg; Total Carbs 26.7g; Fiber 4.9 g; Sugar 18.7 g; Protein 2.9 g

Kiwi Smoothie

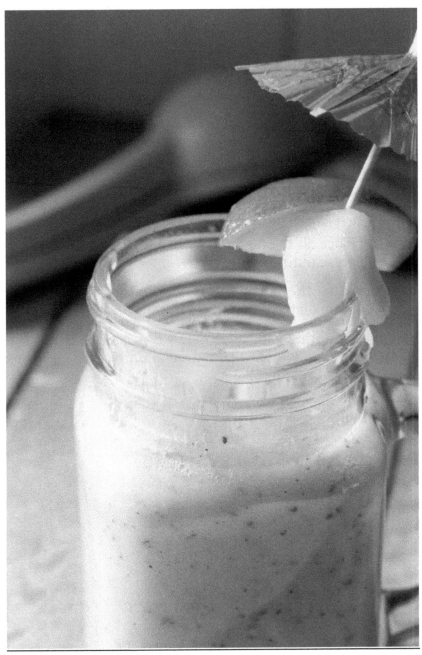

Preparation   Time   :   10   minutes
Cooking Time : 0 minutes

Servings : 2

Ingredients :

- 4 kiwis

- 2 small bananas, peeled

- 1½ cups unsweetened almond milk

- 1-2 drops liquid stevia

- ¼ cup ice cubes

Directions :

1. Place all the ingredients in a high-speed blender and pulse until creamy.

2. Pour the smoothie into two glasses and serve immediately.

Nutrition : Calories 228 Total Fat; 3.8 g Saturated Fat 0.4 g; Cholesterol 0 mg; Sodium 141 mg; Total Carbs 50.7 g; Fiber 8.4 g; Sugar 28.1 g; Protein 3.8 g

Pineapple & Carrot Smoothie

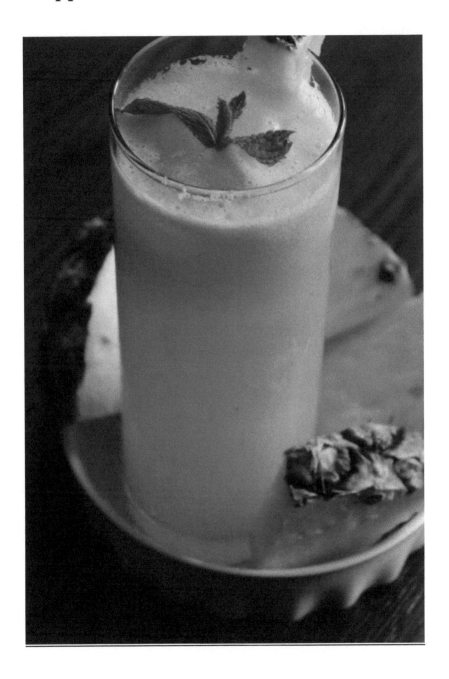

Preparation   Time   :   10   minutes
Cooking Time : 0 minutes

Servings : 2

Ingredients :

- 1 cup frozen pineapple
- 1 large ripe banana, peeled and sliced
- ½ tablespoon fresh ginger, peeled and chopped
- ¼ teaspoon ground turmeric
- 1 cup unsweetened almond milk
- ½ cup fresh carrot juice
- 1 tablespoon fresh lemon juice

Directions :

1. Place all the ingredients in a high-speed blender and pulse until creamy.
2. Pour the smoothie into two glasses and serve immediately.

Nutrition : Calories 132; Total Fat 2.2 g; Saturated Fat 0.3 g; Cholesterol 0 mg; Sodium 113 mg; Total Carbs 629.3 g; Fiber 4.1 g; Sugar 16.9 g; Protein 2 g;

Oats & Orange Smoothie

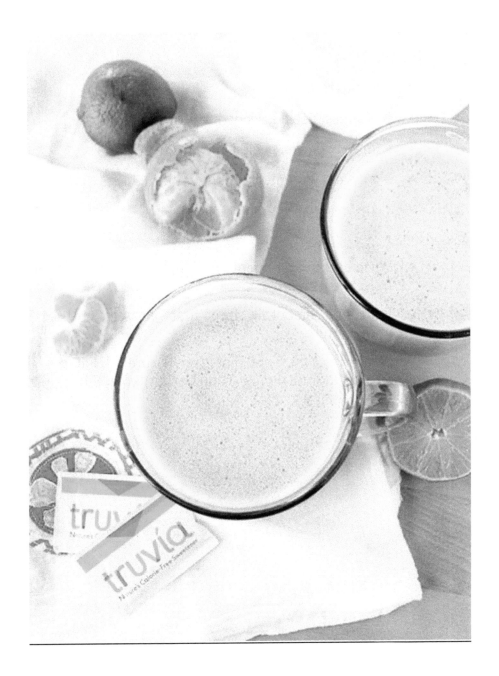

Preparation   Time   :   10   minutes
Cooking Time **:** 0 minutes

Servings **:** 4

Ingredients **:**

- 2/3 cup rolled oats

- 2 oranges, peeled, seeded, and sectioned

- 2 large bananas, peeled and sliced

- 2 cups unsweetened almond milk

- 1 cup ice cubes, crushed

Directions **:**

1. Place all the ingredients in a high-speed blender and pulse until creamy.

2. Pour the smoothie into four glasses and serve immediately.

Nutrition **:** Calories 175; Total Fat 3 g; Saturated Fat 0.4 g; Cholesterol 0 mg; Sodium 93 mg; Total Carbs 36.6 g; Fiber 5.9 g, Sugar 17.1 g, Protein 3.9 g;

Pumpkin Smoothie

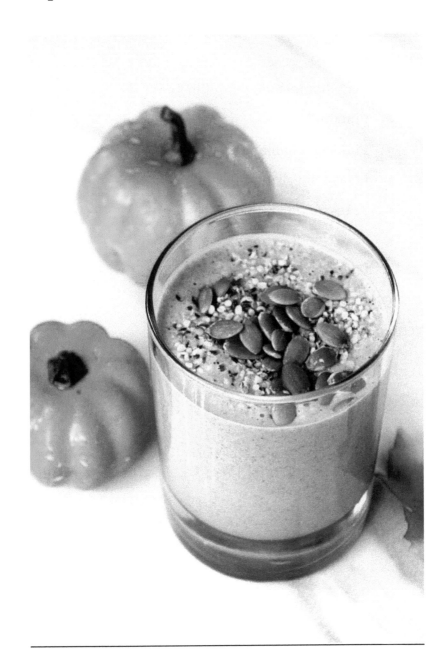

Preparation Time : 10 minutes
Cooking Time : 0 minutes

Servings : 2

Ingredients :

- 1 cup homemade pumpkin puree
- 1 medium banana, peeled and sliced
- 1 tablespoon maple syrup
- 1 teaspoon ground flaxseeds
- ½ teaspoon ground cinnamon
- ¼ teaspoon ground ginger
- 1½ cups unsweetened almond milk
- ¼ cup ice cubes

Directions :

1. Place all the ingredients in a high-speed blender and pulse until creamy.

2. Pour the smoothie into two glasses and serve immediately.

Nutrition : Calories 159; Total Fat 3.6 g; Saturated Fat 0.5 g; Cholesterol 0 mg; Sodium 143 mg; Total Carbs 32.6 g; Fiber 6.5 g, Sugar 17.3 g; Protein 3 g

Red Veggie & Fruit Smoothie

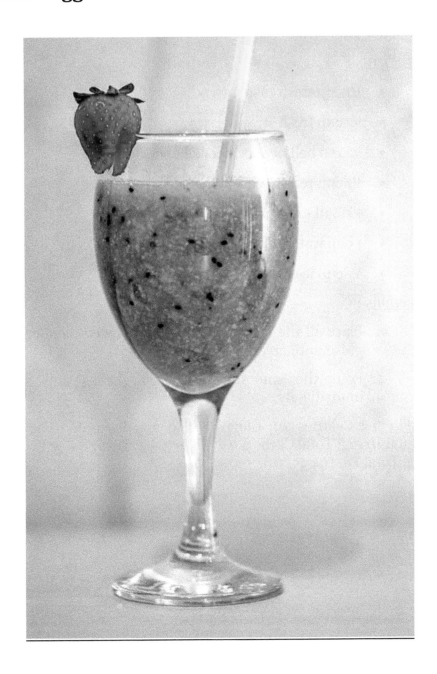

Preparation Time : 10 minutes
Cooking Time : 0 minutes

Servings : 2

Ingredients :

- ½ cup fresh raspberries
- ½ cup fresh strawberries
- ½ red bell pepper, seeded and chopped
- ½ cup red cabbage, chopped
- 1 small tomato
- 1 cup water
- ½ cup ice cubes

Directions :

1. Place all the ingredients in a high-speed blender and pulse until creamy.
2. Pour the smoothie into two glasses and serve immediately.

Nutrition : Calories 39; Cholesterol 0 mg; Saturated Fat 0 g; Sodium 10 mg; Total Carbs 8.9 g; Fiber 3.5 g; Sugar 4.8 g; Protein 1.3 g, Total Fat 0.4 g

Dandelion Avocado Smoothie

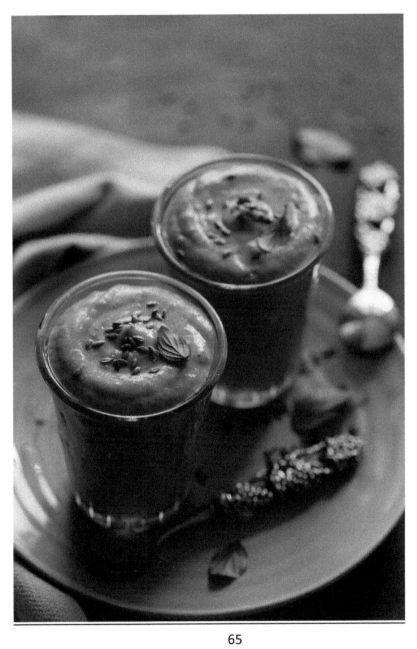

Preparation Time : 15 minutes

Cooking Time : 0

Servings : 1

Ingredients :

- One cup of Dandelion
- One Orange (juiced)
- Coconut water
- One Avocado
- One key lime (juice)

Directions :

1. In a high-speed blender until smooth, blend Ingredients.

Nutrition : Calories: 160; Fat: 15 g; Carbohydrates: 9 g; Protein: 2 g

Amaranth Greens and Avocado Smoothie

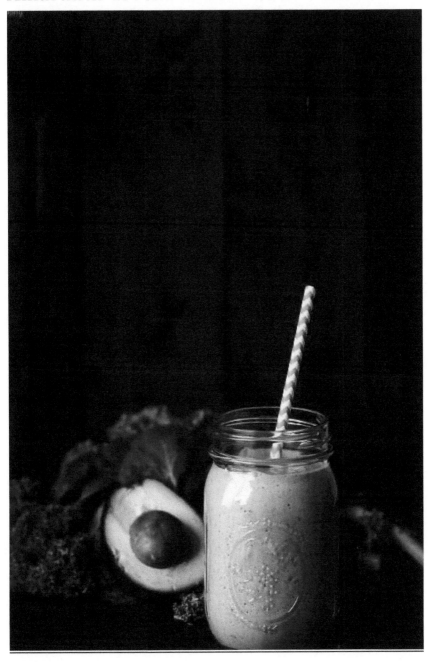

Preparation Time : 15 minutes

Cooking Time : 0

Servings : 1

Ingredients :

- One key lime (juice).
- Two sliced apples (seeded).
- Half avocado.
- Two cupsful of amaranth greens.
- Two cupsful of watercress.
- One cupful of water.

Directions :

1. Add the whole recipes together and transfer them into the blender. Blend thoroughly until smooth.

Nutrition : Calories: 160; Fat: 15 g; Carbohydrates: 9 g; Protein: 2 g

Lettuce, Orange and Banana Smoothie

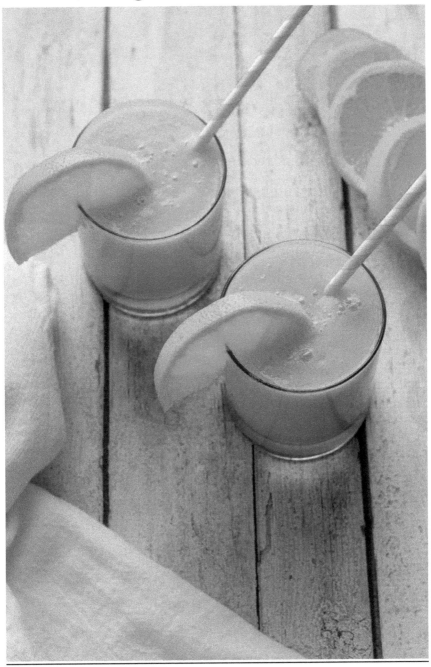

Preparation Time : 15 minutes

Cooking Time : 0

Servings : 1

Ingredients :

- One and a half cupsful of fresh lettuce.
- One large banana.
- One cup of mixed berries of your choice.
- One juiced orange.

Directions :

1. First, add the orange juice to your blender.
2. Add the remaining recipes and blend thoroughly.
3. Enjoy the rest of your day.

Nutrition : Calories: 252.1; Protein: 4.1 g

Delicious Elderberry Smoothie

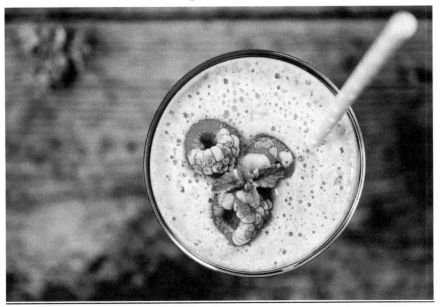

Preparation Time : 15 minutes

Cooking Time : 0

Servings : 1

Ingredients :

- One cupful of Elderberry
- One cupful of Cucumber
- One large apple
- A quarter cupful of water

Directions :

1. Add the whole recipes together into a blender. Grind very well until they are uniformly smooth and enjoy.

Nutrition : Calories: 106; Carbohydrates: 26.68

Peaches Zucchini Smoothie

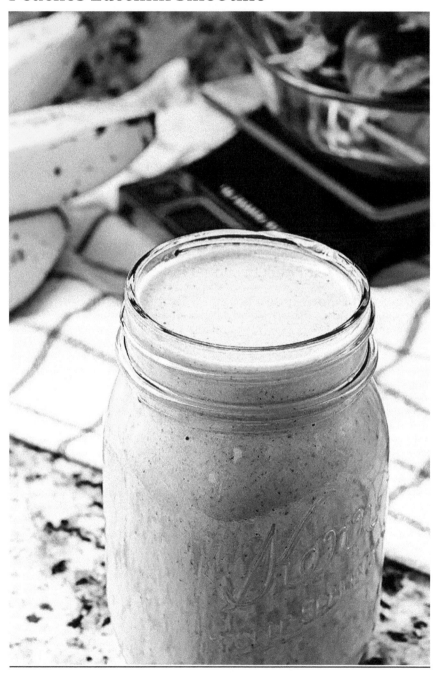

Preparation Time : 15 minutes

Cooking Time : 0

Servings : 1

Ingredients :

- A half cupful of squash.

- A half cupful of peaches.

- A quarter cupful of coconut water.

- A half cupful of Zucchini.

Directions :

1. Add the whole recipes together into a blender and blend until smooth and serve.

Nutrition : 55 Calories; 0g Fat; 2g Of Protein; 10mg Sodium; 14 G Carbohydrate; 2g Of Fiber

Ginger Orange and Strawberry Smoothie

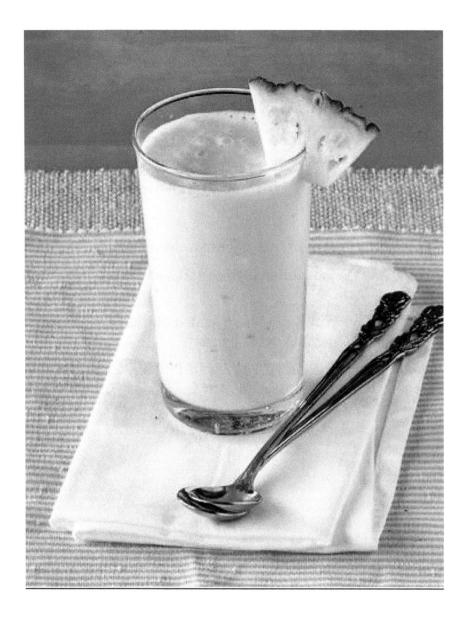

Preparation Time : 15 minutes

Cooking Time : 0

Servings : 1

Ingredients :

- One cup of strawberry.

- One large orange (juice)

- One large banana.

- Quarter small sized ginger (peeled and sliced).

Directions :

2. Transfer the orange juice to a clean blender.

3. Add the remaining recipes and blend thoroughly until smooth.

4. Enjoy. Wow! You have ended the 9th day of your weight loss and detox journey.

Nutrition : 32 Calories; 0.3g Fat; 2g Of Protein; 10mg Sodium; 14g Carbohydrate; Water; 2g Of Fiber.

Kale Parsley and Chia Seeds Detox Smoothie

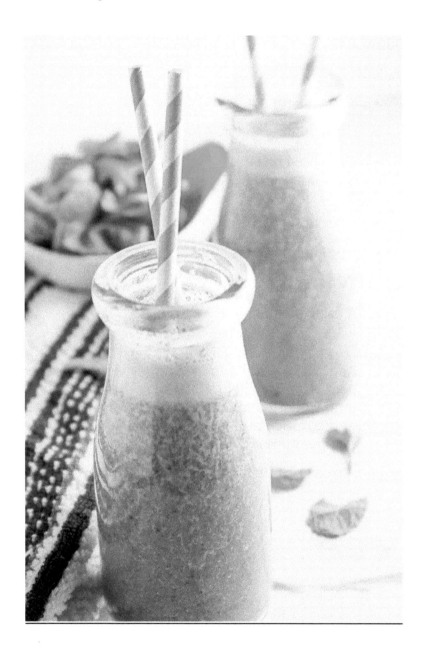

Preparation Time : 15 minutes

Cooking Time : 0

Servings : 1

Ingredients :

- Three tbsp. chia seeds (grounded).
- One cupful of water.
- One sliced banana.
- One pear (chopped).
- One cupful of organic kale.
- One cupful of parsley.
- Two tbsp. of lemon juice.
- A dash of cinnamon.

Directions :

1. Add the whole recipes together into a blender and pour the water before blending. Blend at high speed until smooth and enjoy. You may or may not place it in the refrigerator depending on how hot or cold the weather appears.

Nutrition : 75 calories; 1g fat; 5g protein; 10g fiber

Watermelon Limenade

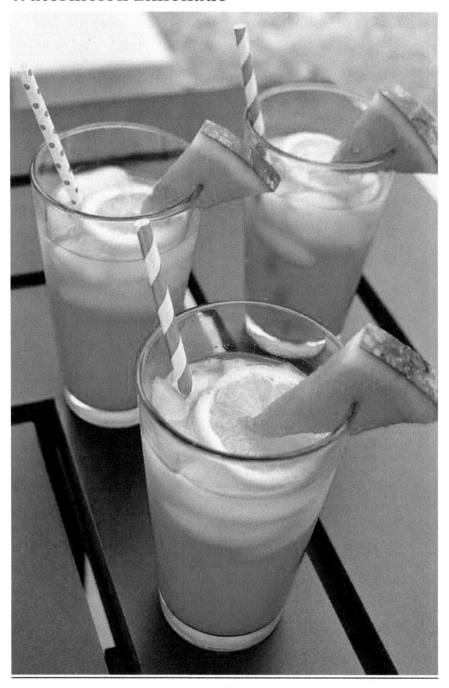

Preparation Time : 5 Minutes

Cooking Time : 0 minutes

Servings : 6

When it comes to refreshing summertime drinks, lemonade is always near the top of the list. This Watermelon "Limenade" is perfect for using up leftover watermelon or for those early fall days when stores and farmers are almost giving them away. You can also substitute 4 cups of ice for the cold water to create a delicious summertime slushy.

Ingredients:

- 4 cups diced watermelon
- 4 cups cold water
- 2 tablespoons freshly squeezed lemon juice
- 1 tablespoon freshly squeezed lime juice

Directions:

1. In a blender, combine the watermelon, water, lemon juice, and lime juice, and blend for 1 minute.

2. Strain the contents through a fine-mesh sieve or nut-milk bag. Serve chilled. Store in the refrigerator for up to 3 days.

SERVING TIP: Slice up a few lemon or lime wedges to serve with your Watermelon Limenade, or top it with a few fresh mint leaves to give it an extra-crisp, minty flavor.

Nutrition : Calories: 60

Bubbly Orange Soda

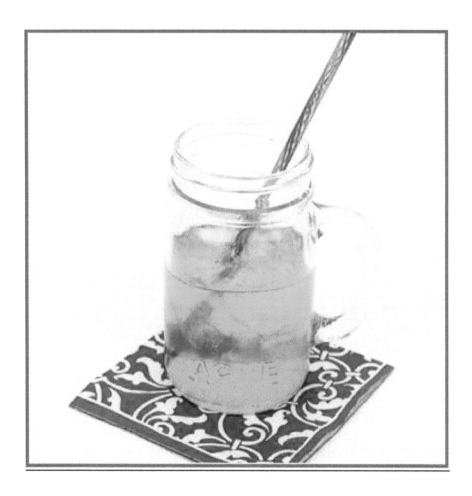

Preparation Time : 5 Minutes

Cooking Time : 0 minutes

Servings : 4

Soda can be one of the toughest things to give up when you first adopt a WFPB diet. That's partially because refined sugars and caffeine are addictive, but it can also be because carbonated beverages are fun to drink! With sweetness from the orange juice and bubbliness from the carbonated water, this orange "soda" is perfect for assisting in the transition from SAD to WFPB.

Ingredients:

- 4 cups carbonated water

- 2 cups pulp-free orange juice (4 oranges, freshly squeezed and strained)

Directions:

1. For each serving, pour 2 parts carbonated water and 1-part orange juice over ice right before serving.

2. Stir and enjoy.

SERVING TIP: This recipe is best made right before drinking. The amount of fizz in the carbonated water will decrease the longer it's open, so if you're going to make it ahead of time, make sure it's stored in an airtight, refrigerator-safe container.

Nutrition: Calories: 56

Creamy Cashew Milk

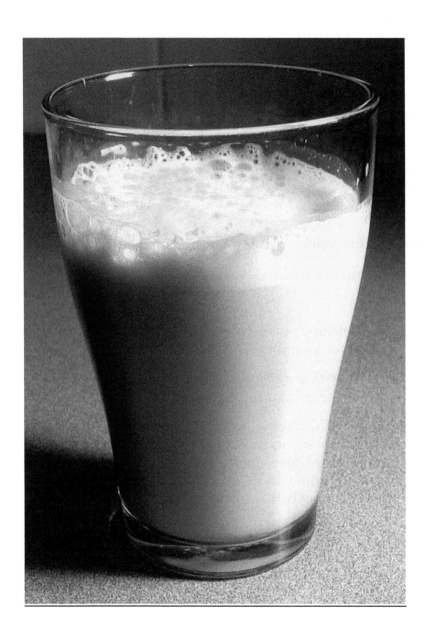

Preparation Time : 5 Minutes

Cooking Time : 0 minutes

Servings : 8

Learning how to make your own plant-based milks can be one of the best ways to save money and ditch dairy for good. This is one of the easiest milk recipes to master, and if you have a high-speed blender, you can skip the straining step and go straight to a refrigerator-safe container. Large mason jars work great for storing plant-based milk, as they allow you to give a quick shake before each use.

Ingredients:

- 4 cups water

- ¼ cup raw cashews, soaked overnight

Directions:

1. In a blender, blend the water and cashews on high speed for 2 minutes.

2. Strain with a nut-milk bag or cheesecloth, then store in the refrigerator for up to 5 days.

VARIATION TIP: This recipe makes unsweetened cashew milk that can be used in savory and sweet dishes. For a creamier version to put in your coffee, cut the amount of water in half. For a sweeter version, add 1 to 2 tablespoons maple syrup and 1 teaspoon vanilla extract before blending.

Nutrition: Calories: 18

Homemade Oat Milk

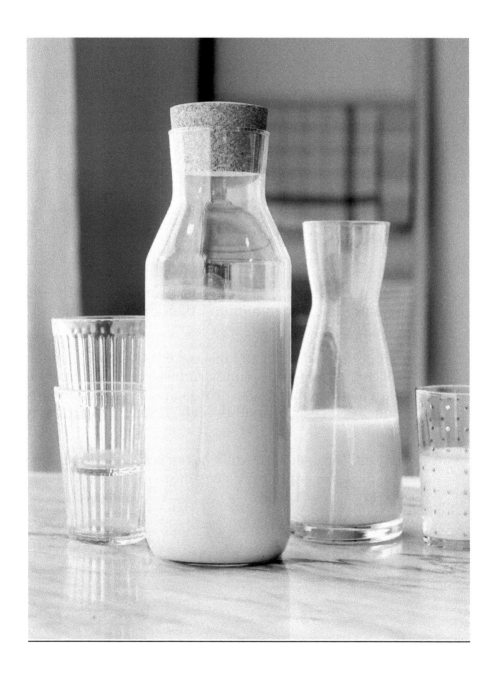

Preparation Time : 5 Minutes

Cooking Time : 0 minutes

Servings : 8

Oat milk is a fantastic option if you need a nut-free milk or just want an extremely inexpensive plant-based milk. Making a half-gallon jar at home costs a fraction of the price of other plant-based or dairy milks. Oat milk can be used in both savory and sweet dishes.

Ingredients:

- 1 cup rolled oats

- 4 cups water

Directions:

1. Put the oats in a medium bowl, and cover with cold water. Soak for 15 minutes, then drain and rinse the oats.

2. Pour the cold water and the soaked oats into a blender. Blend for 60 to 90 seconds, or just until the mixture is a creamy white color throughout. (Blending any further may over blend the oats, resulting in a gummy milk.)

3. Strain through a nut-milk bag or colander, then store in the refrigerator for up to 5 days.

Nutrition: Calories: 39

Lucky Mint Smoothie

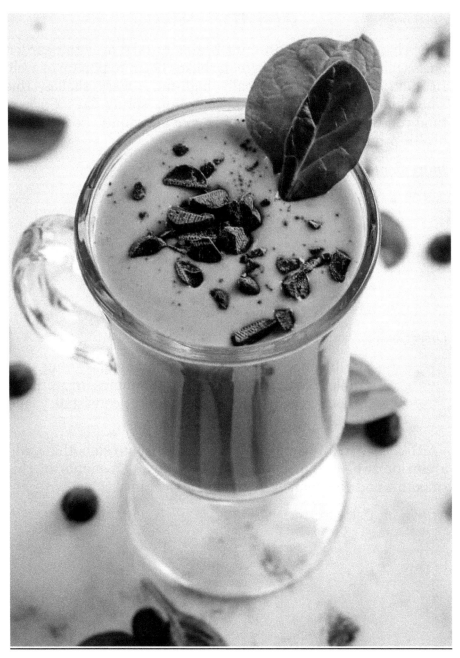

Preparation Time : 5 Minutes

Cooking Time : 0 minutes

Servings : 2

As spring approaches and mint begins to take over the garden once again, "Irish"-themed green shakes begin to pop up as well. In contrast to the traditionally high-fat, sugary shakes, this smoothie is a wonderful option for sunny spring days. So next time you want to sip on something cool and minty, do so with a health-promoting Lucky Mint Smoothie.

Ingredients:

- 2 cups plant-based milk (here or here)

- 2 frozen bananas, halved

- 1 tablespoon fresh mint leaves or ¼ teaspoon peppermint extract

- 1 teaspoon vanilla extract

Directions :

1. In a blender, combine the milk, bananas, mint, and vanilla. Blend on high for 1 to 2 minutes, or until the contents reach a smooth and creamy consistency, and serve.

VARIATION TIP: If you like to sneak greens into smoothies, add a cup or two of spinach to boost the health benefits of this smoothie and give it an even greener appearance.

Nutrition: Calories: 152

Paradise Island Smoothie

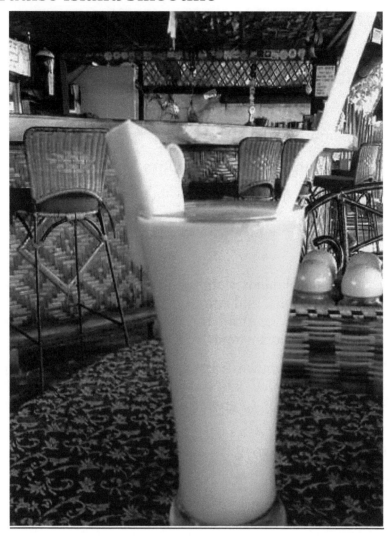

Preparation Time : 5 Minutes

Cooking Time : 0 minutes

Servings : 2

Ingredients :

- 2 cups plant-based milk (here or here)
- 1 frozen banana
- ½ cup frozen mango chunks
- ½ cup frozen pineapple chunks
- 1 teaspoon vanilla extract

Directions :

1. In a blender, combine the milk, banana, mango, pineapple, and vanilla. Blend on high for 1 to 2 minutes, or until the contents reach a smooth and creamy consistency, and serve.

LEFTOVER TIP: If you have any leftover smoothie, you can put it in a jar with some rolled oats and allow the mixture to soak in the refrigerator overnight to create a tropical version of overnight oats.

Nutrition: Calories: 176

Apple Pie Smoothie

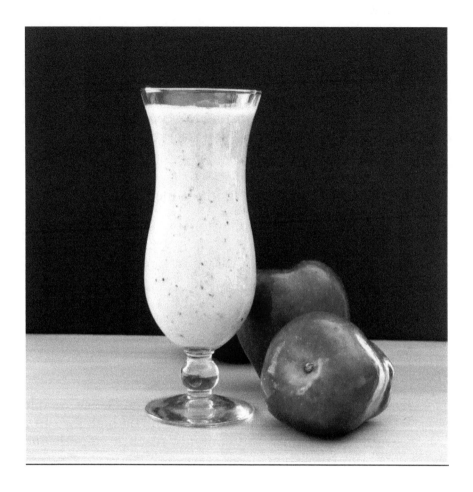

Preparation Time : 5 Minutes

Cooking Time : 0 minutes

Servings : 2

This smoothie is great for a quick breakfast or a cool dessert. Its combination of sweet apples and warming cinnamon is sure to win over children and adults alike. If the holidays find you in a warm area, this smoothie may just be the cool treat you've been looking for to take the place of pie at dessert time.

Ingredients:

- 2 sweet crisp apples, cut into 1-inch cubes
- 2 cups plant-based milk (here or here)
- 1 cup ice
- 1 tablespoon maple syrup
- 1 teaspoon ground cinnamon
- 1 teaspoon vanilla extract

Directions:

1. In a blender, combine the apples, milk, ice, maple syrup, cinnamon, and vanilla. Blend on high for 1 to 2 minutes, or until the contents reach a smooth and creamy consistency, and serve.

VARIATION TIP: You can also use this recipe for making overnight oatmeal. Blend your smoothie, mix it with 2 cups rolled oats, and refrigerate overnight for a premade breakfast for two.

Nutrition: Calories: 198

Choco-Nut Milkshake

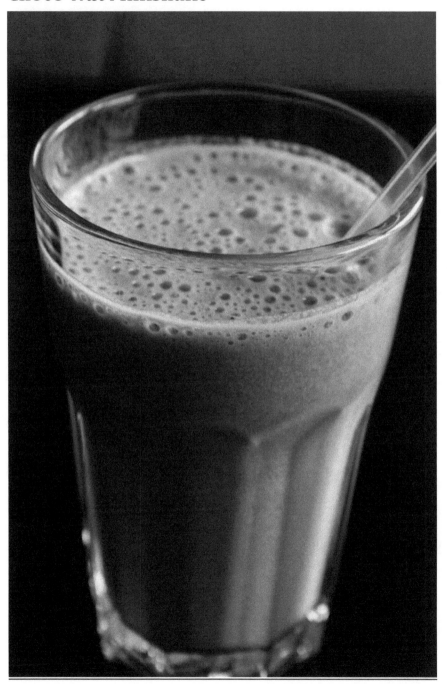

Preparation Time : 10 minutes

Cooking Time : 0 minute

Serving : 2

Ingredients:

- 2 cups unsweetened coconut, almond
- 1 banana, sliced and frozen
- ¼ cup unsweetened coconut flakes
- 1 cup ice cubes
- ¼ cup macadamia nuts, chopped
- 3 tablespoons sugar-free sweetener
- 2 tablespoons raw unsweetened cocoa powder
- Whipped coconut cream

Directions :

1. Place all ingredients into a blender and blend on high until smooth and creamy.
2. Divide evenly between 4 "mocktail" glasses and top with whipped coconut cream, if desired.
3. Add a cocktail umbrella and toasted coconut for added flair.
4. Enjoy your delicious Choco-nut smoothie!

Nutrition: 12g Carbohydrates; 3g Protein; 199 Calories

Pineapple & Strawberry Smoothie

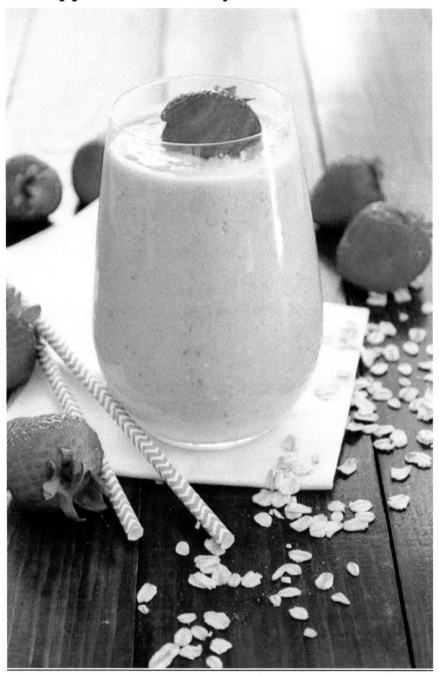

Preparation Time : 7 minutes

Cooking Time : 0 minute

Serving : 2

Ingredients :

- 1 cup strawberries
- 1 cup pineapple, chopped
- ¾ cup almond milk
- 1 tablespoon almond butter

Directions :

1. Add all ingredients to a blender.
2. Blend until smooth.
3. Add more almond milk until it reaches your desired consistency.
4. Chill before serving.

Nutrition : 255 Calories; 39g Carbohydrate; 5.6g Protein

Cantaloupe Smoothie

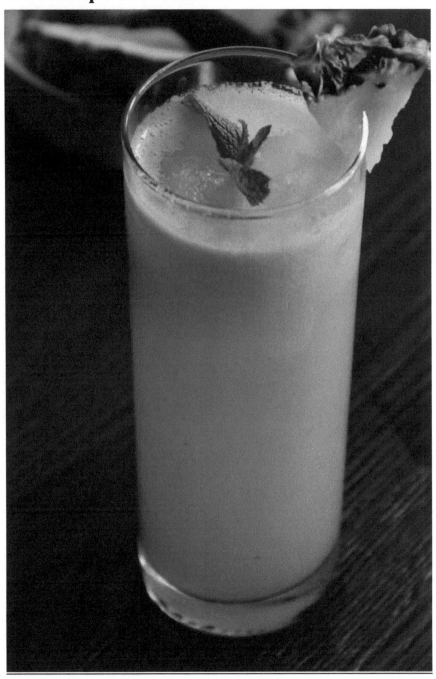

Preparation Time : 11 minutes

Cooking Time : 0 minute

Serving : 2

Ingredients :

- ¾ cup carrot juice
- 4 cups cantaloupe, sliced into cubes
- Pinch of salt
- Frozen melon balls
- Fresh basil

Directions :

1. Add the carrot juice and cantaloupe cubes to a blender. Sprinkle with salt.
2. Process until smooth.
3. Transfer to a bowl.
4. Chill in the refrigerator for at least 30 minutes.
5. Top with the frozen melon balls and basil before serving.

Nutrition : 135 Calories; 31g Carbohydrate; 3.4g Protein

Berry Smoothie with Mint

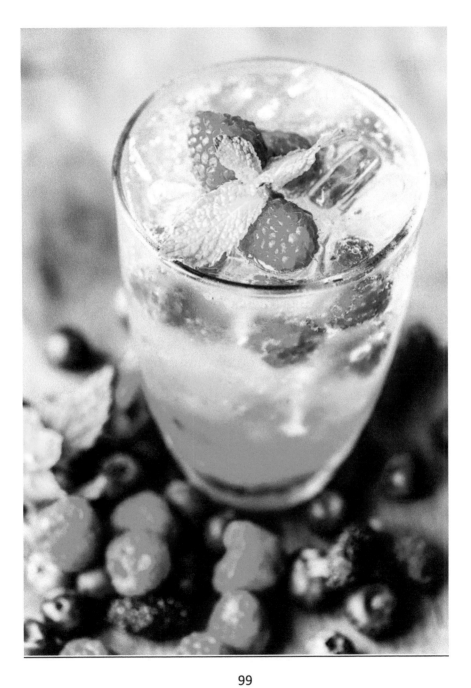

Preparation Time : 7 minutes

Cooking Time : 0 minute

Serving : 2

Ingredients :

- ¼ cup orange juice
- ½ cup blueberries
- ½ cup blackberries
- 1 cup reduced-fat plain kefir
- 1 tablespoon honey
- 2 tablespoons fresh mint leaves

Directions :

1. Add all the ingredients to a blender.
2. Blend until smooth.

Nutrition : 137 Calories; 27g Carbohydrate; 6g Protein

Green Smoothie

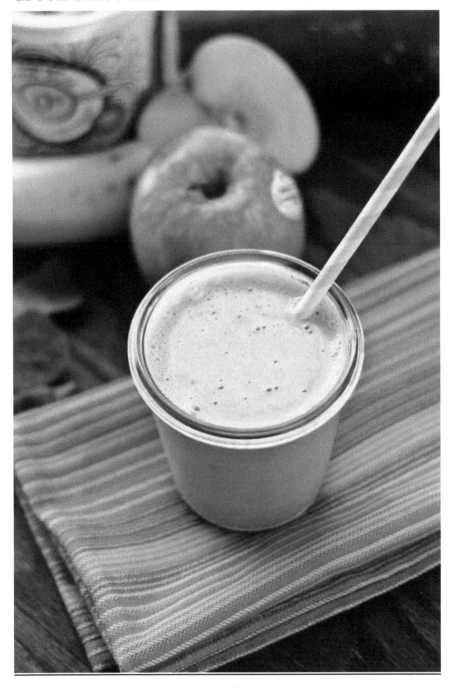

Preparation Time : 12 minutes

Cooking Time : 0 minute

Serving : 2

Ingredients :

- 1 cup vanilla almond milk (unsweetened)
- ¼ ripe avocado, chopped
- 1 cup kale, chopped
- 1 banana
- 2 teaspoons honey
- 1 tablespoon chia seeds
- 1 cup ice cubes

Directions :

1. Combine all the ingredients in a blender.
2. Process until creamy.

Nutrition : 343 Calories; 14.7g Carbohydrate; 5.9g Protein

Banana, Cauliflower & Berry Smoothie

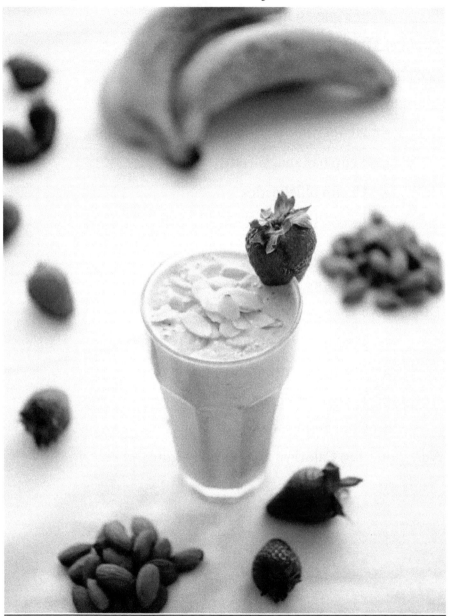

Preparation Time : 9 minutes

Cooking Time : 0 minute

Serving : 2

Ingredients :

- 2 cups almond milk (unsweetened)
- 1 cup banana, sliced
- ½ cup blueberries
- ½ cup blackberries
- 1 cup cauliflower rice
- 2 teaspoons maple syrup

Directions :

1. Pour almond milk into a blender.
2. Stir in the rest of the ingredients.
3. Process until smooth.
4. Chill before serving.

Nutrition : 149 Calories; 29g Carbohydrate; 3g Protein

Berry & Spinach Smoothie

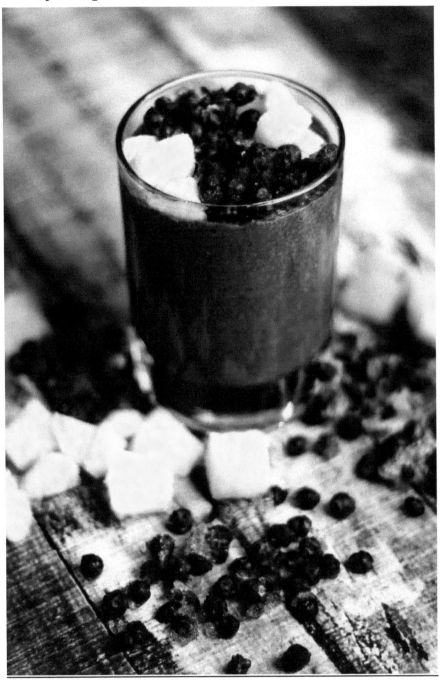

Preparation Time : 11 minutes

Cooking Time : 0 minute

Serving : 2

Ingredients :

- 2 cups strawberries
- 1 cup raspberries
- 1 cup blueberries
- 1 cup fresh baby spinach leaves
- 1 cup pomegranate juice
- 3 tablespoons milk powder (unsweetened)

Directions :

1. Mix all the ingredients in a blender.
2. Blend until smooth.
3. Chill before serving.

Nutrition : 118 Calories; 25.7g Carbohydrate; 4.6g Protein

Peanut Butter Smoothie with Blueberries

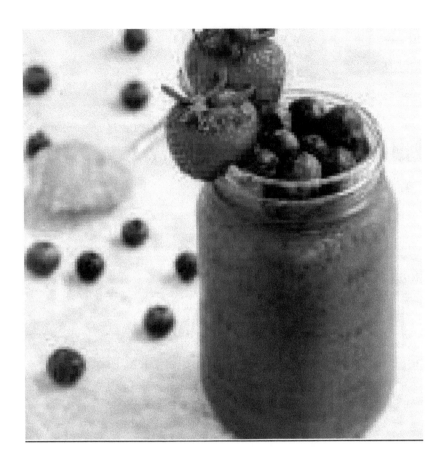

Preparation Time : 12 minutes

Cooking Time : 0 minute

Serving : 2

Ingredients :

- 2 tablespoons creamy peanut butter
- 1 cup vanilla almond milk (unsweetened)
- 6 oz. soft silken tofu
- ½ cup grape juice
- 1 cup blueberries
- Crushed ice

Directions :

1. Mix all the ingredients in a blender.
2. Process until smooth.

Nutrition : 247 Calories; 30g Carbohydrate; 10.7g Protein

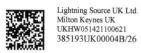

Lightning Source UK Ltd.
Milton Keynes UK
UKHW051421100621
385193UK00004B/26

9 781802 699890